Milky Moments

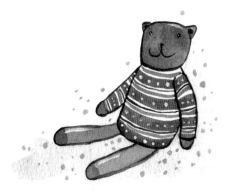

For Hope, our inspiration, and her Granby,
and for Bella
with our love xx

With grateful thanks to everybody who has helped with Milky Moments, especially Marcus Hearn, Scott Barton, Justine Fieth, Ruth Danson, Susannah Fountain, Mel Findlater, Eric Gowland, Jacque Gerrard, Beka Wylie, Kathryn Brown, Clare Josey, Martin Wagner, Zoë Blanc and the many mothers and children who listened to words and looked at illustrations. Thank you, as well, to Roy, Hope's Daddy, for many a scrumptious curry along the way.

To marvellous midwives, and to the many wonderful women who support mothers as they begin and continue to breastfeed, thank you, thank you, thank you. Without one of them, Rachel O'Leary, Ellie and Hope's breastfeeding journey (and therefore this book), might never have begun.

Hope is dancing! Esperanza!

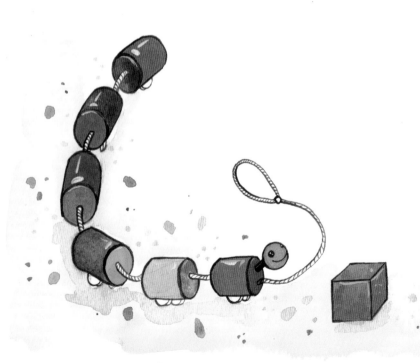

Milky Moments
First published by Pinter & Martin Ltd 2015, reprinted 2018
Text copyright © 2015 Ellie Stoneley
Illustrations copyright © 2015 Ellie Stoneley and Jessica D'Alton Goode
ISBN 978-1-78066-255-8 (hardback)
ISBN 978-1-78066-256-5 (paperback)

British Library Cataloguing-in-Publication Data
A catalogue record for this book is available from the British Library

Printed in Poland by HussarBooks.

Pinter & Martin Ltd
6 Effra Parade
London SW2 1PS

www.pinterandmartin.com

Milky Moments

Ellie Stoneley   illustrated by Jessica D'Alton Goode

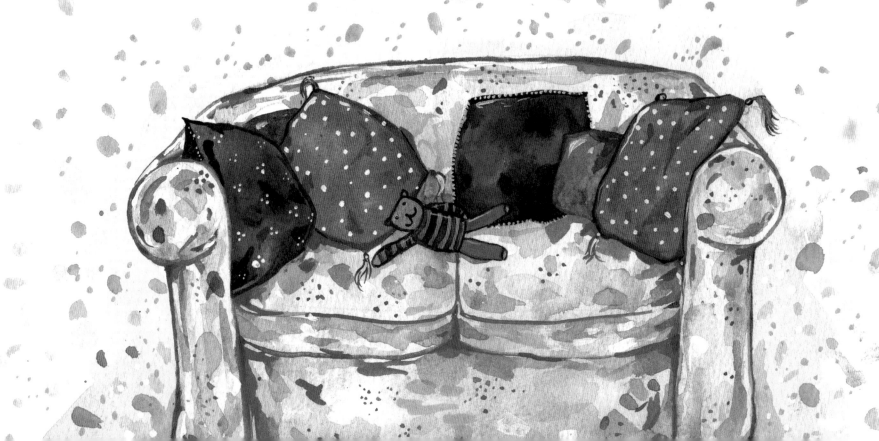

pinter & martin

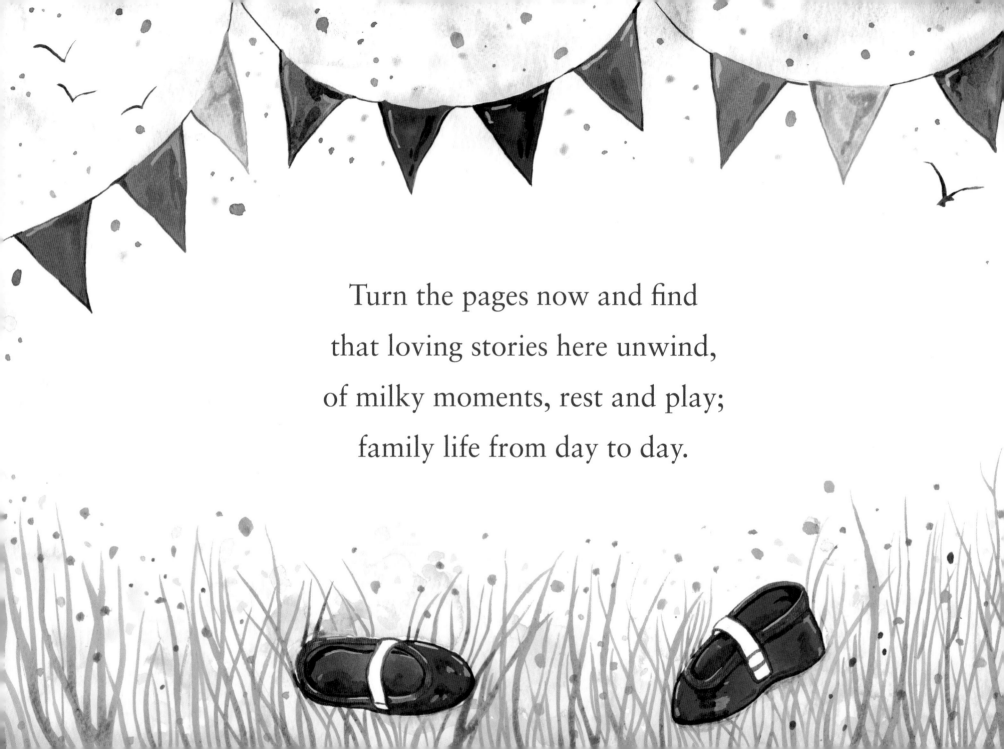

Turn the pages now and find
that loving stories here unwind,
of milky moments, rest and play;
family life from day to day.

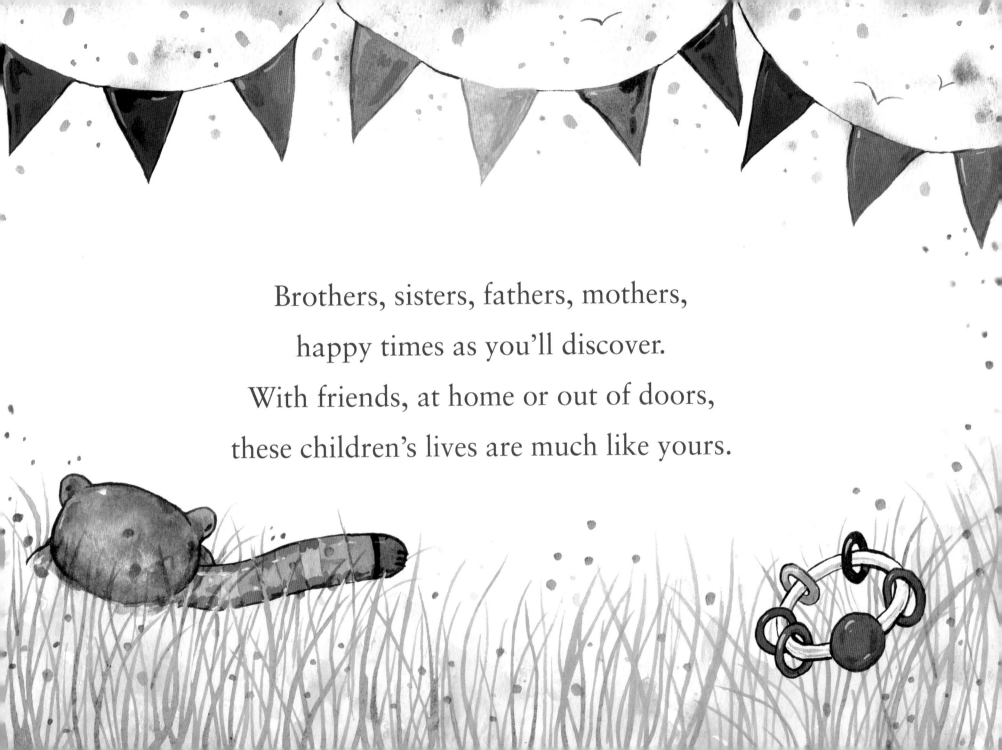

Brothers, sisters, fathers, mothers,
happy times as you'll discover.
With friends, at home or out of doors,
these children's lives are much like yours.

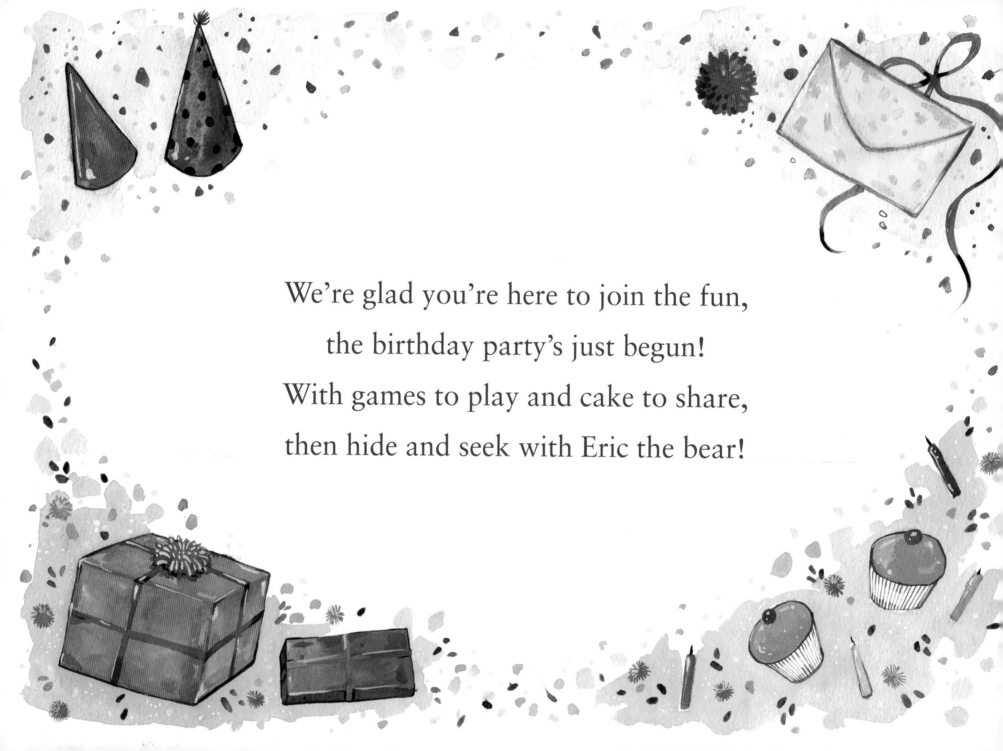

We're glad you're here to join the fun,
the birthday party's just begun!
With games to play and cake to share,
then hide and seek with Eric the bear!

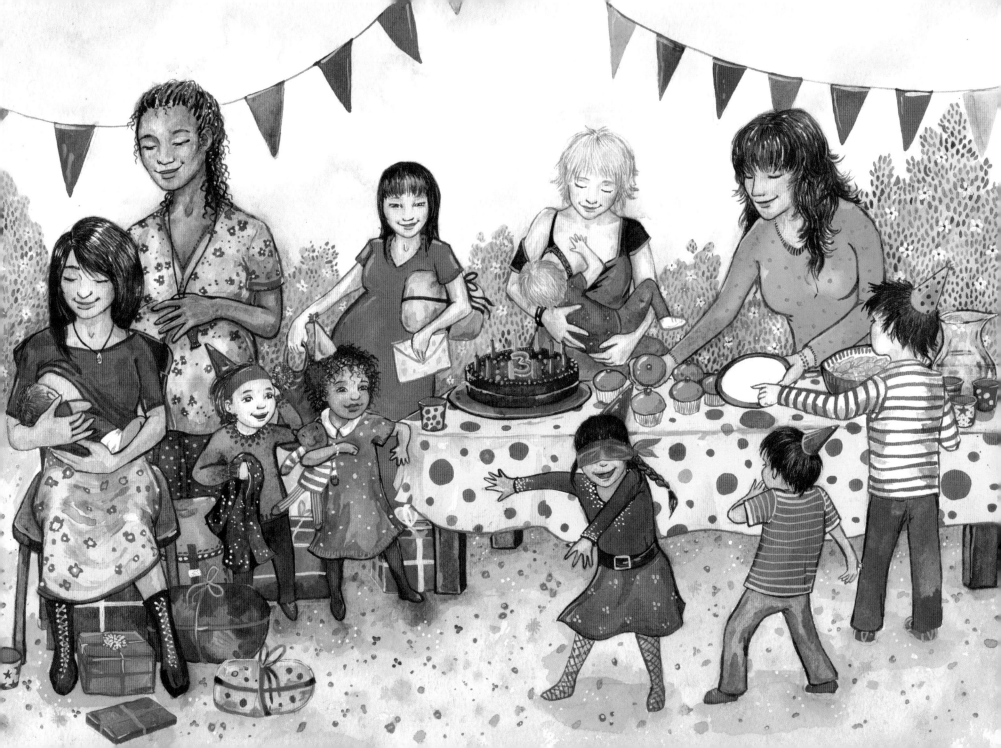

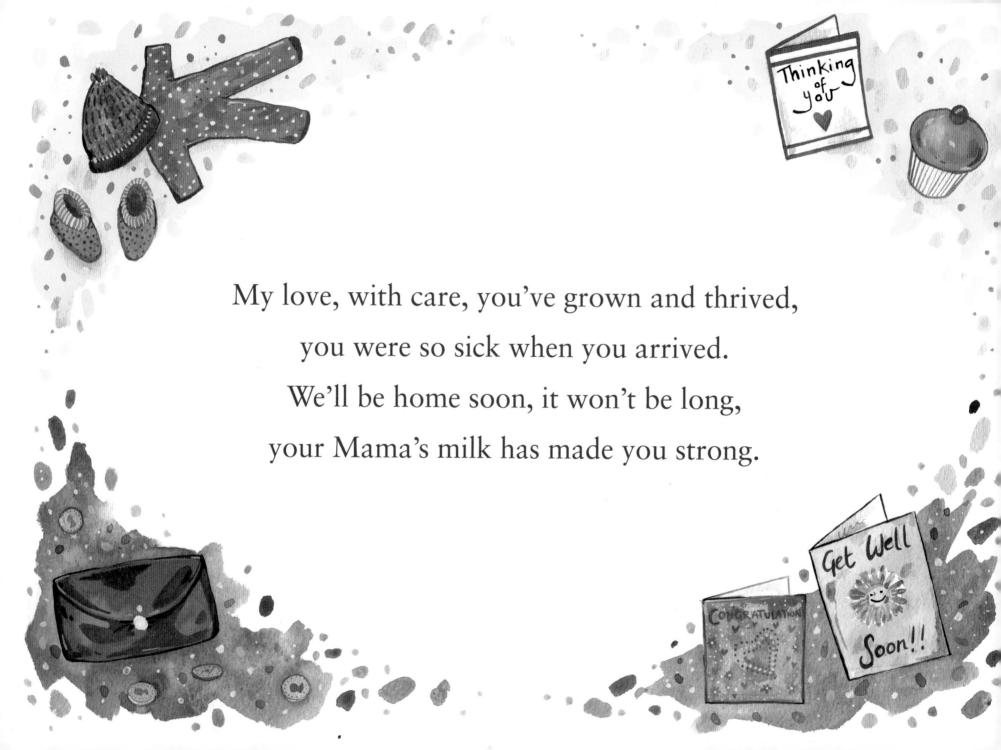

My love, with care, you've grown and thrived,

you were so sick when you arrived.

We'll be home soon, it won't be long,

your Mama's milk has made you strong.

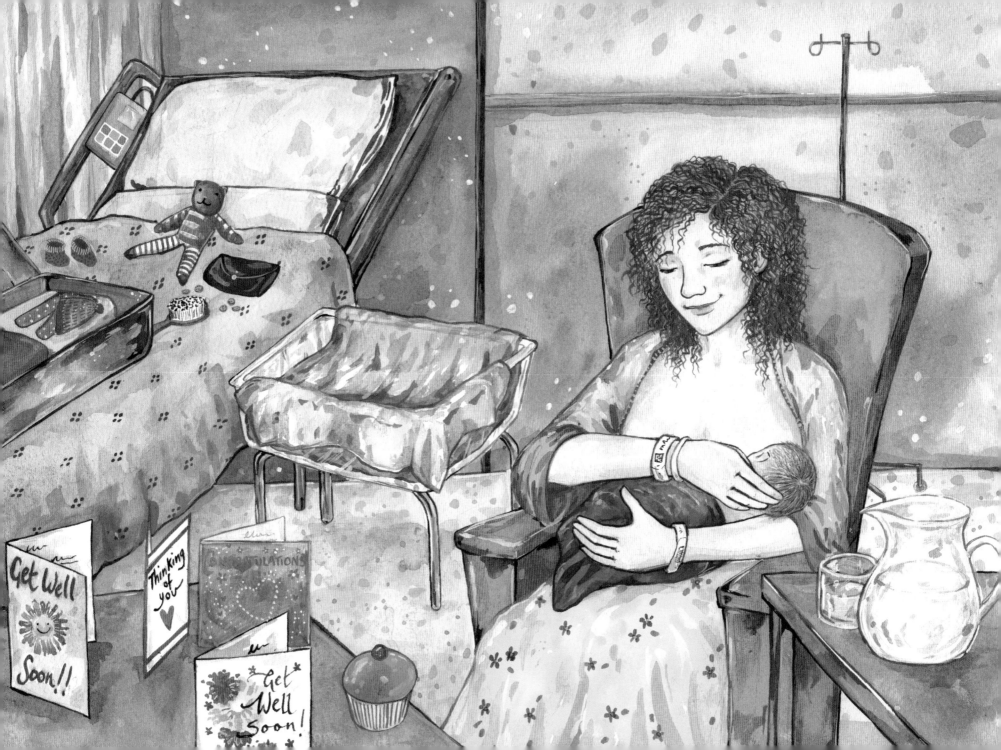

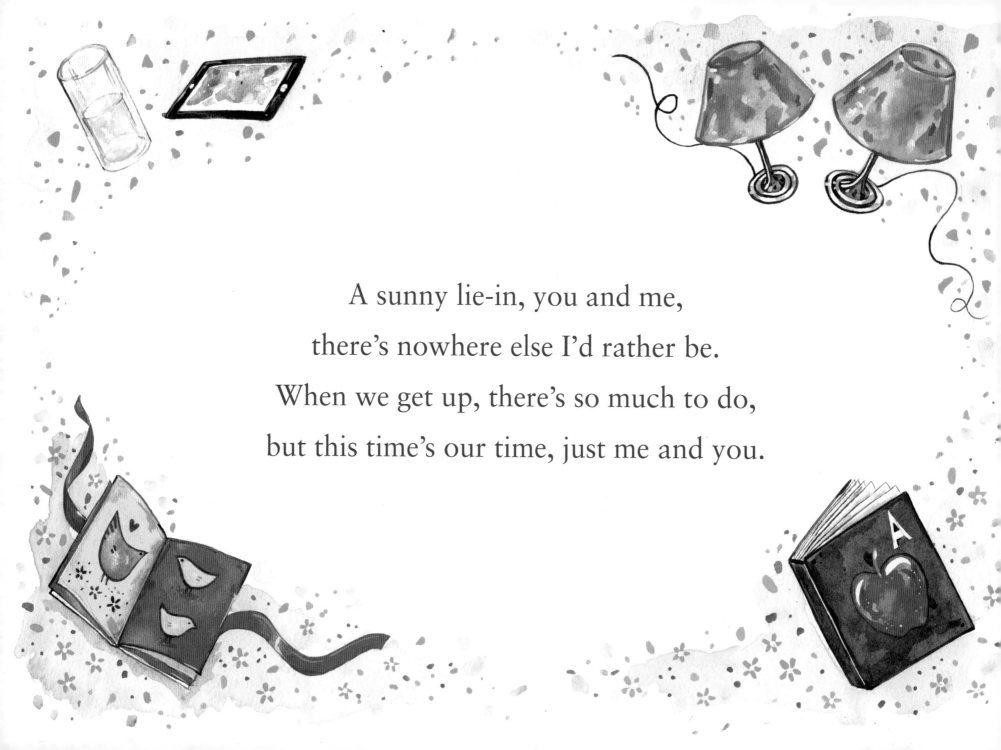

A sunny lie-in, you and me,

there's nowhere else I'd rather be.

When we get up, there's so much to do,

but this time's our time, just me and you.

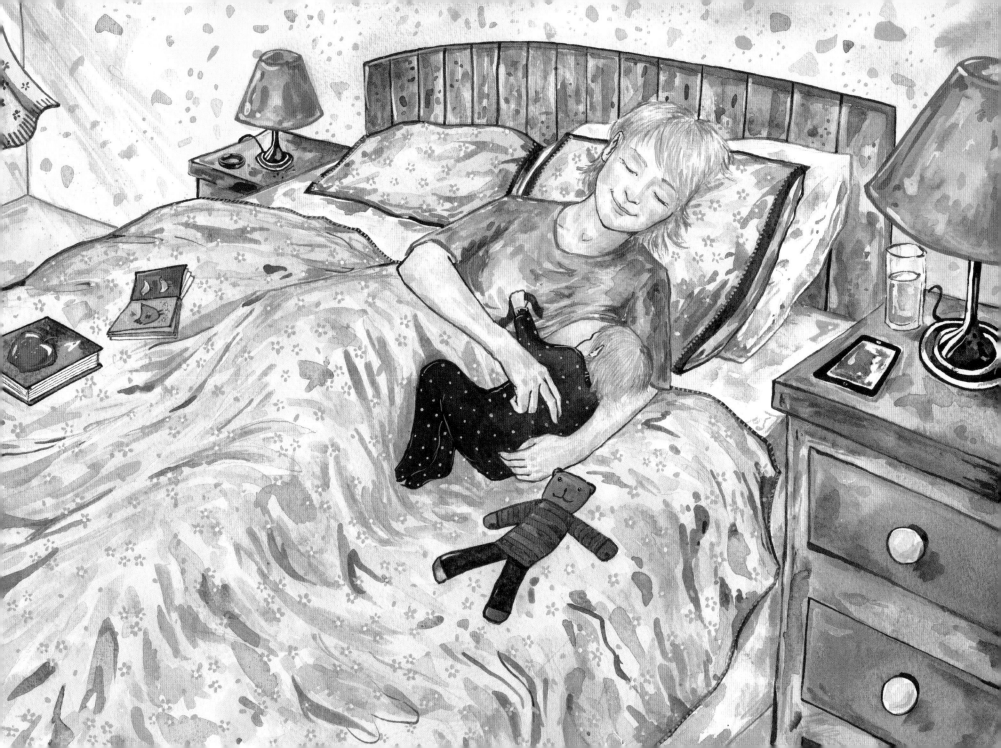

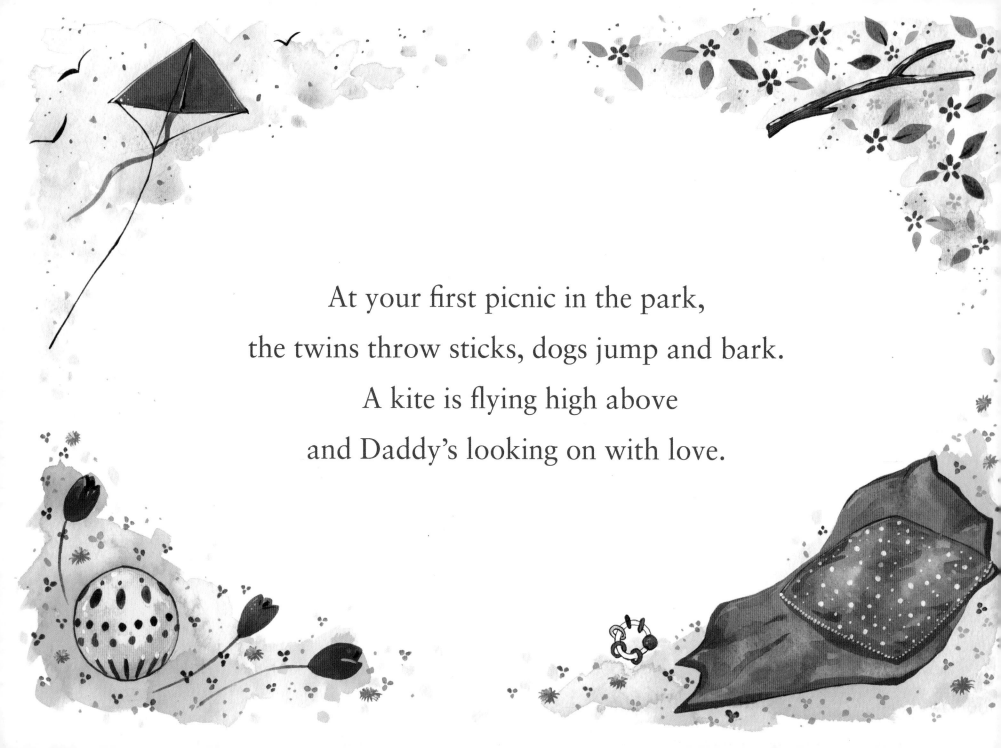

At your first picnic in the park,

the twins throw sticks, dogs jump and bark.

A kite is flying high above

and Daddy's looking on with love.

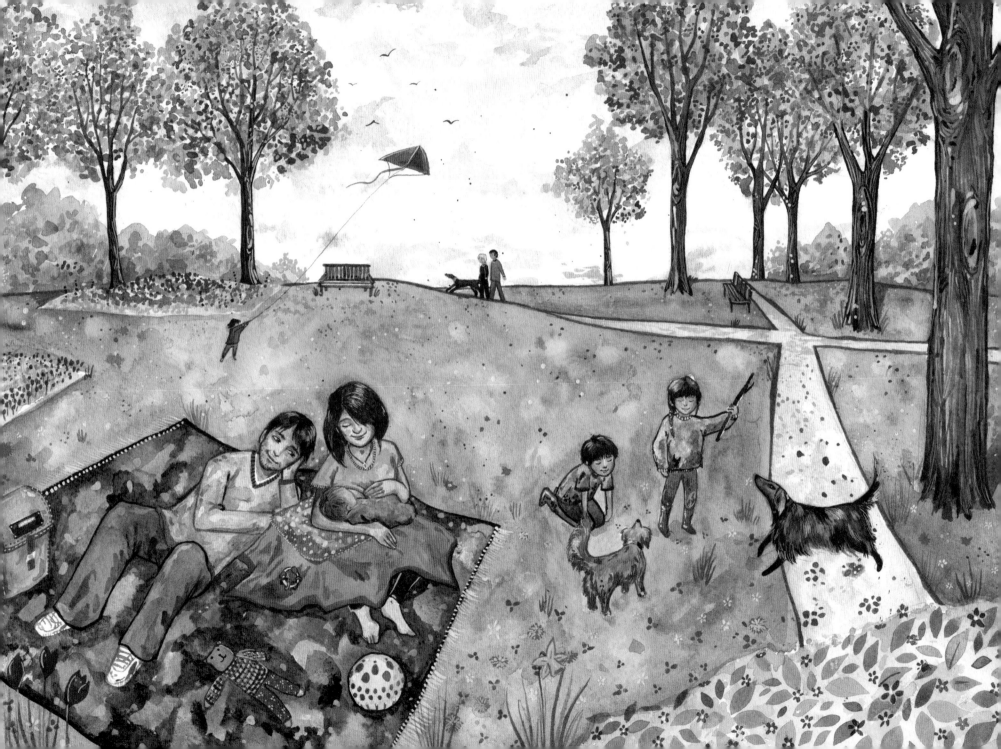

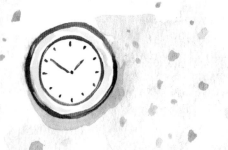

Precious baby, so brand new,

I will always care for you.

I'll hold you close and kiss your head,

with Mama's milk, you'll be well fed.

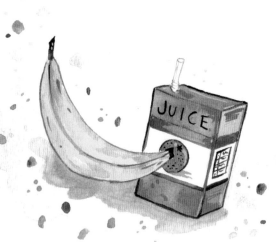
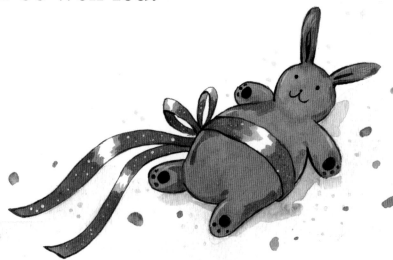

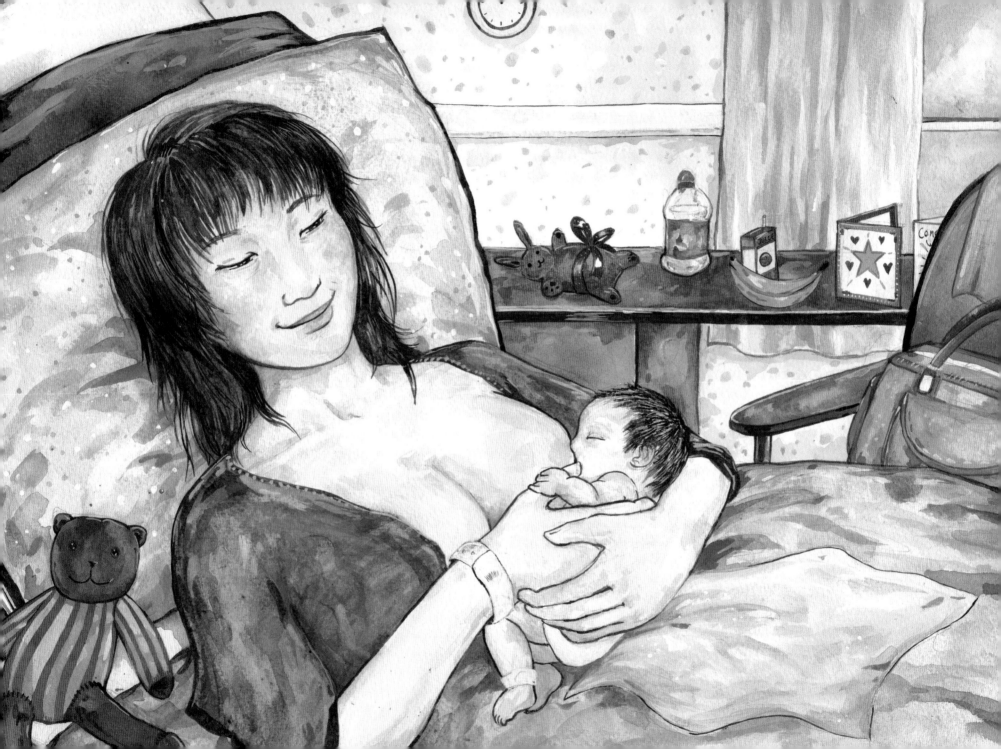

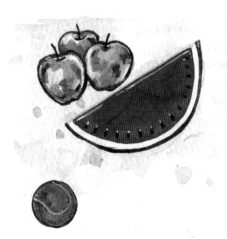

On a bright and breezy summer's day

the beach is a glorious place to play:

sandcastles, shells and a splash in the sea.

Your ice cream is melting! It's dripped on Dad's knee.

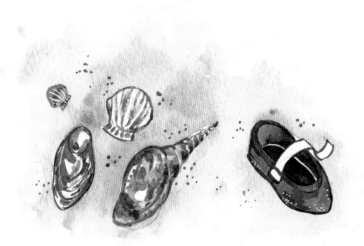

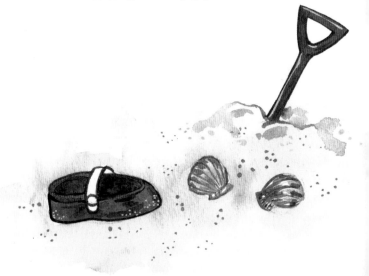

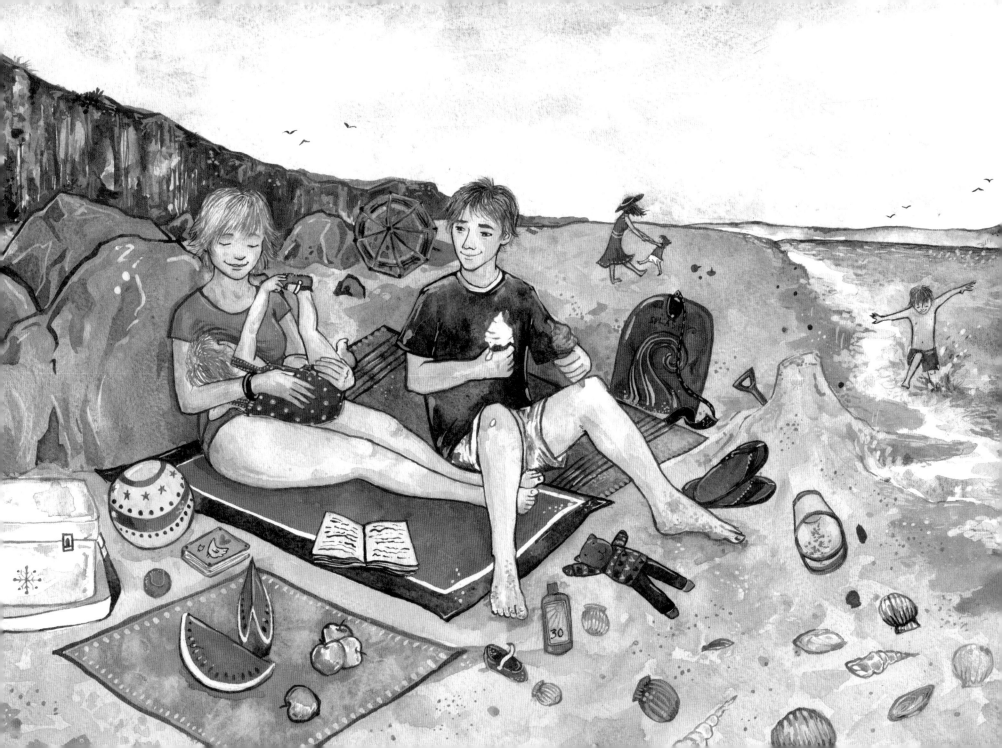

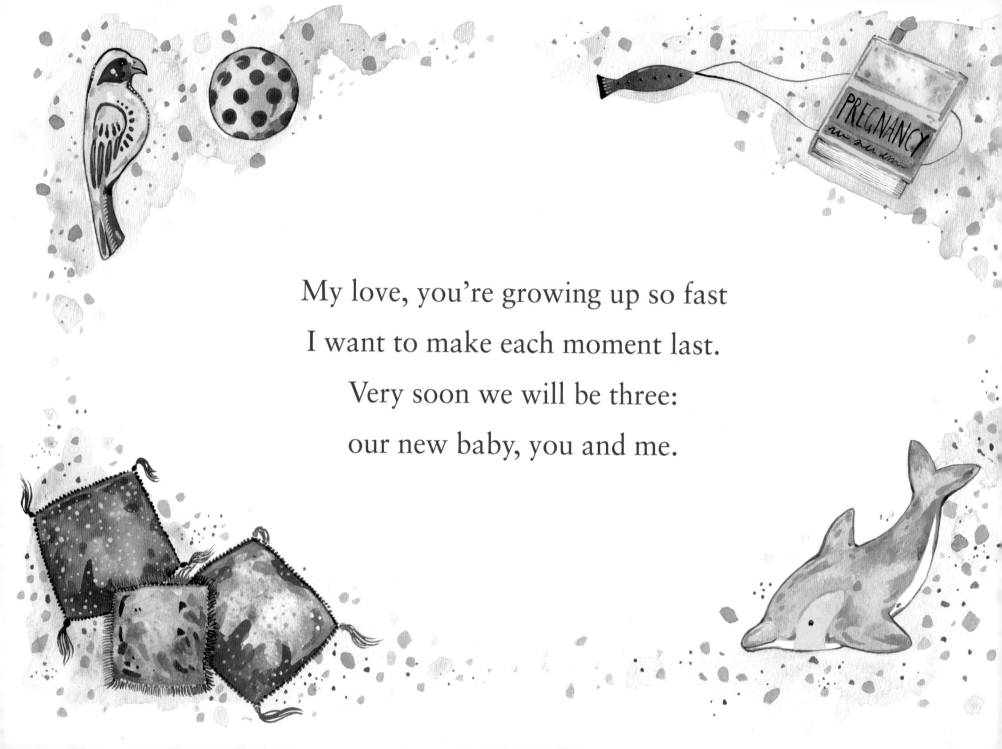

My love, you're growing up so fast

I want to make each moment last.

Very soon we will be three:

our new baby, you and me.

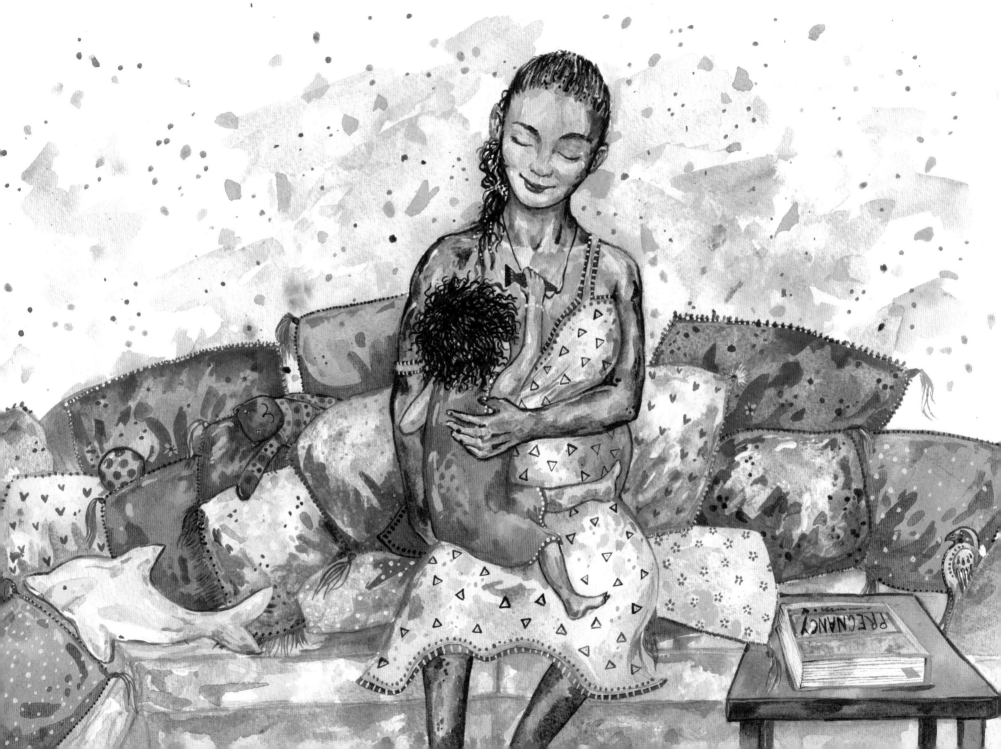

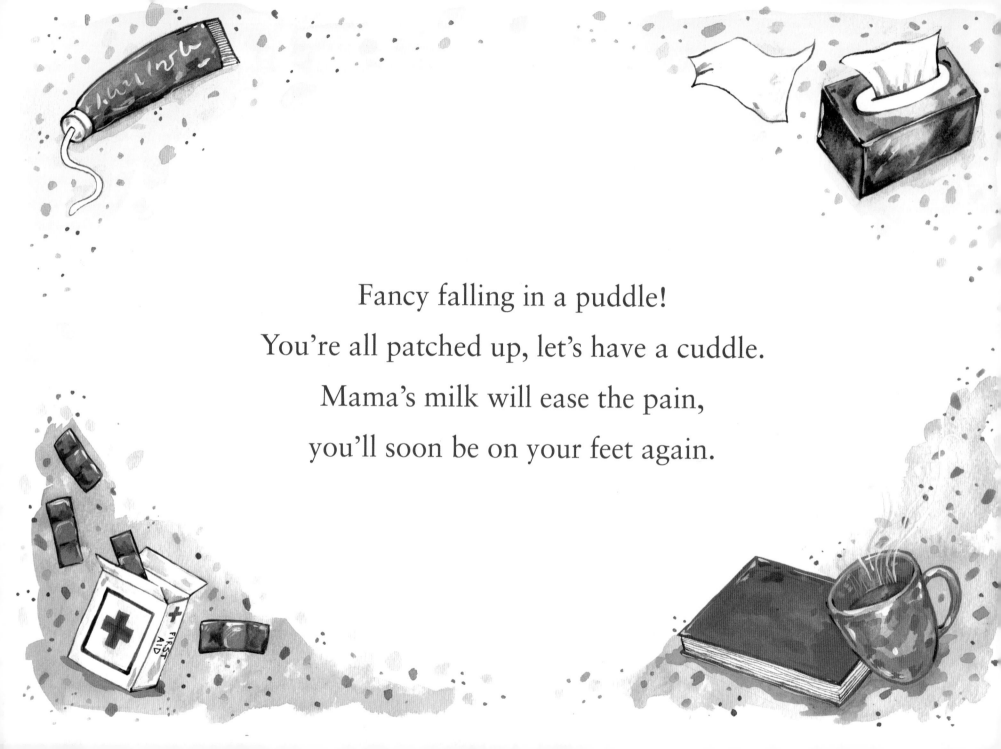

Fancy falling in a puddle!

You're all patched up, let's have a cuddle.

Mama's milk will ease the pain,

you'll soon be on your feet again.

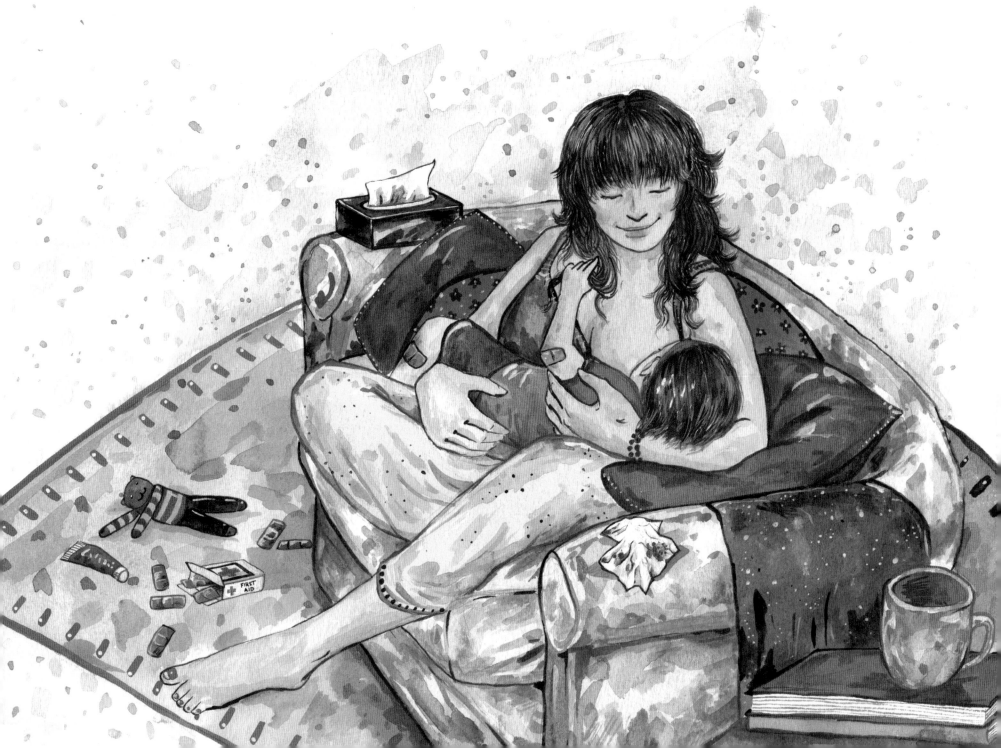

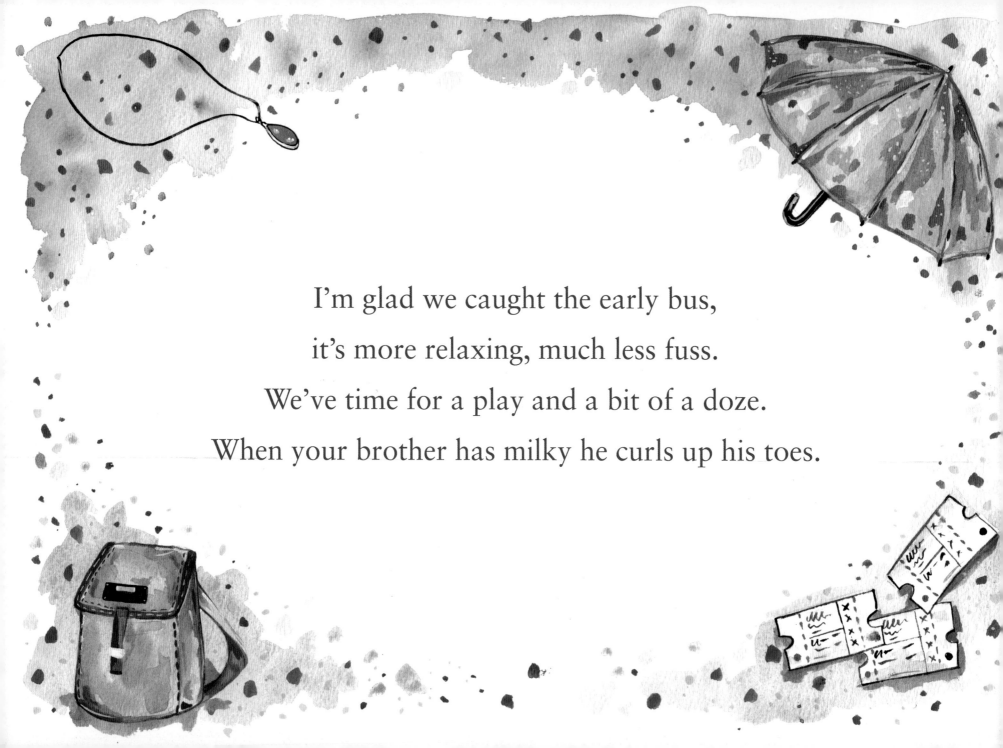

I'm glad we caught the early bus,

it's more relaxing, much less fuss.

We've time for a play and a bit of a doze.

When your brother has milky he curls up his toes.

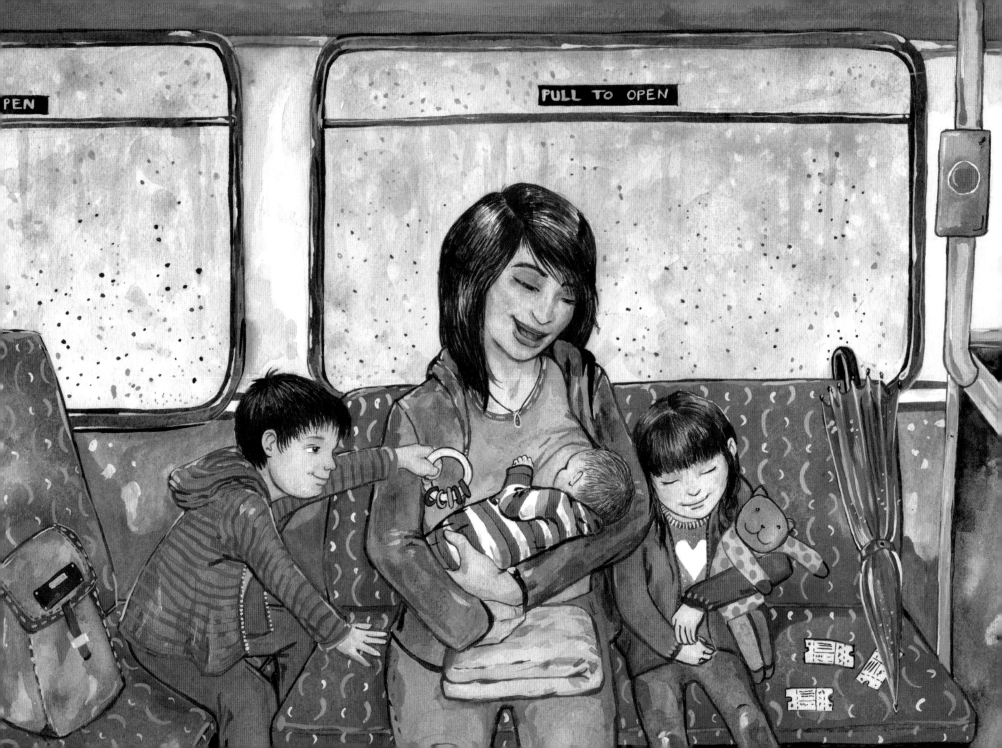

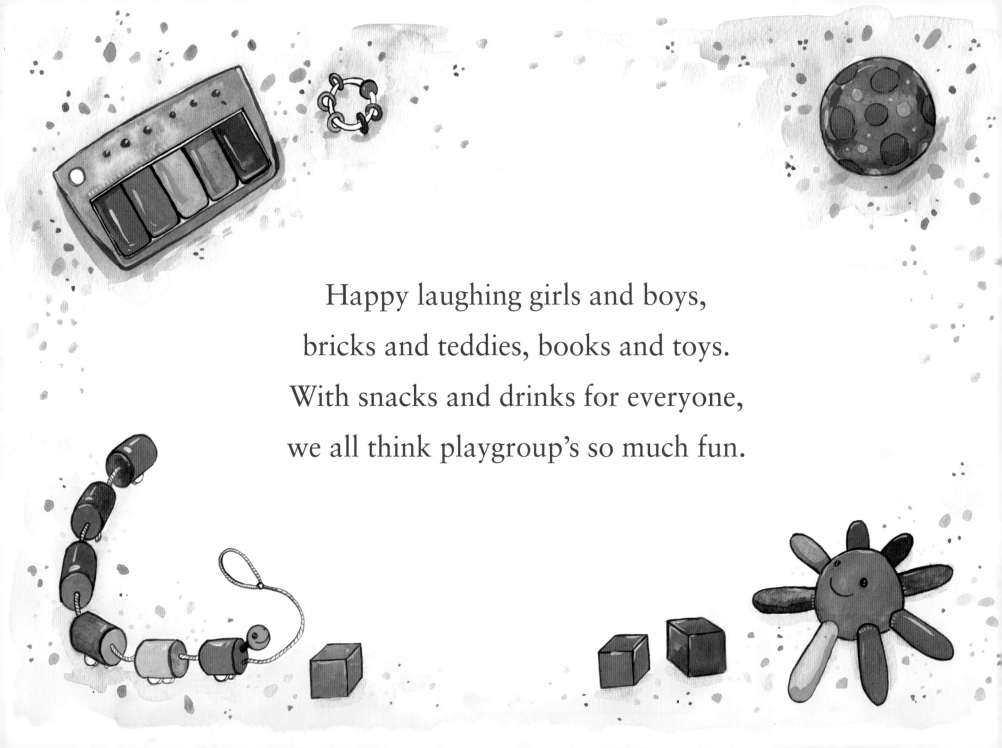

Happy laughing girls and boys,
bricks and teddies, books and toys.
With snacks and drinks for everyone,
we all think playgroup's so much fun.

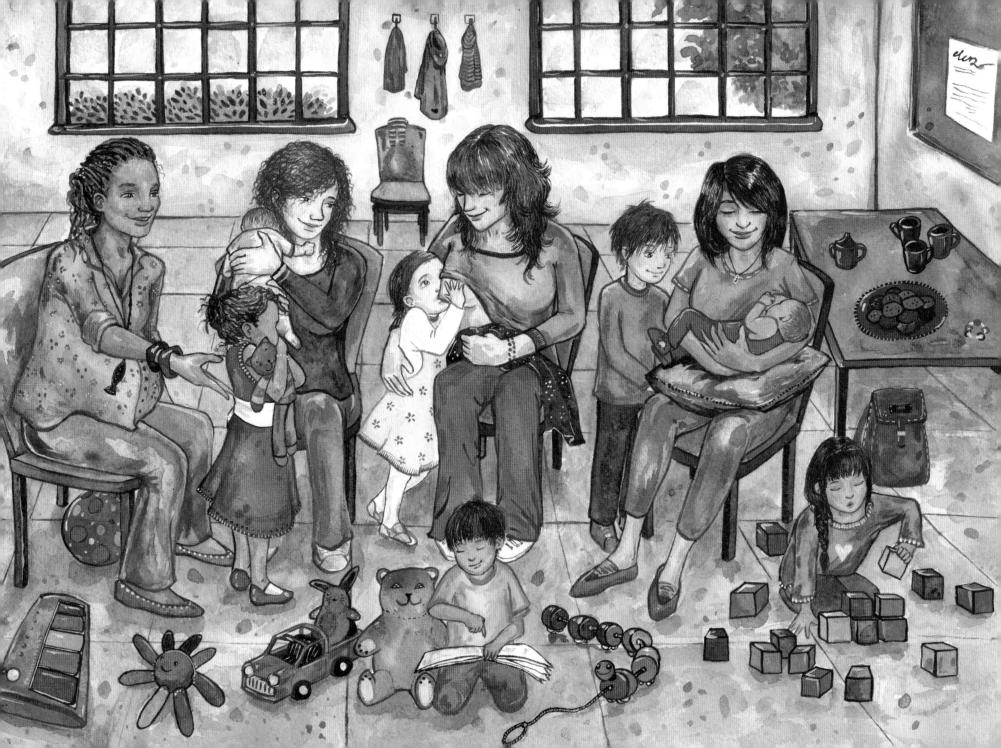

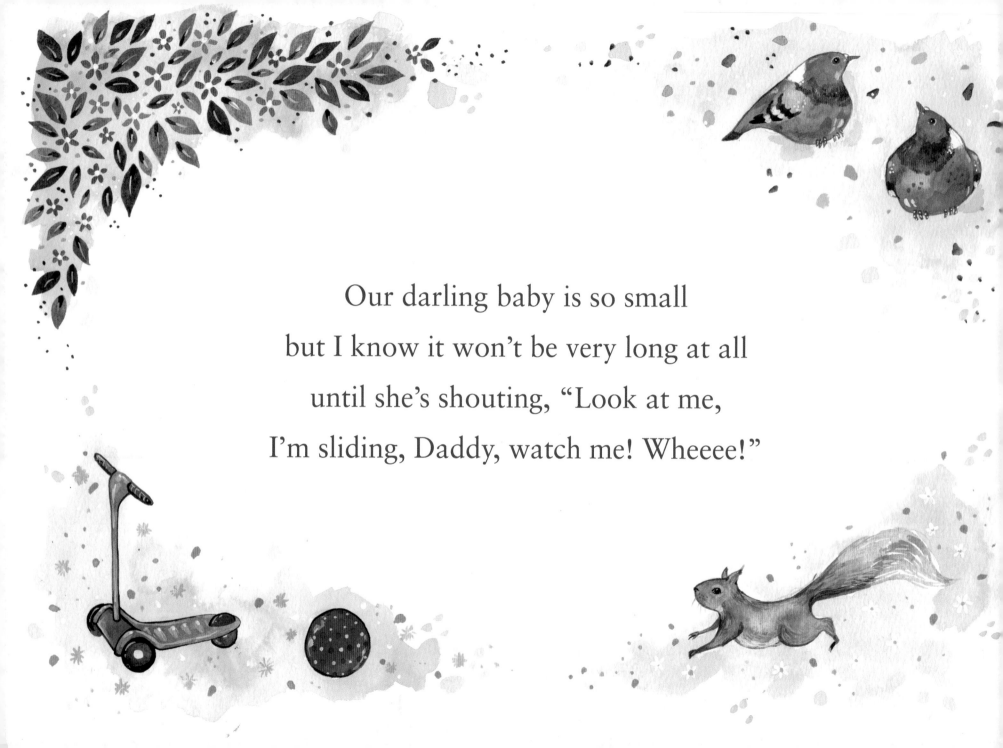

Our darling baby is so small
but I know it won't be very long at all
until she's shouting, "Look at me,
I'm sliding, Daddy, watch me! Wheeee!"

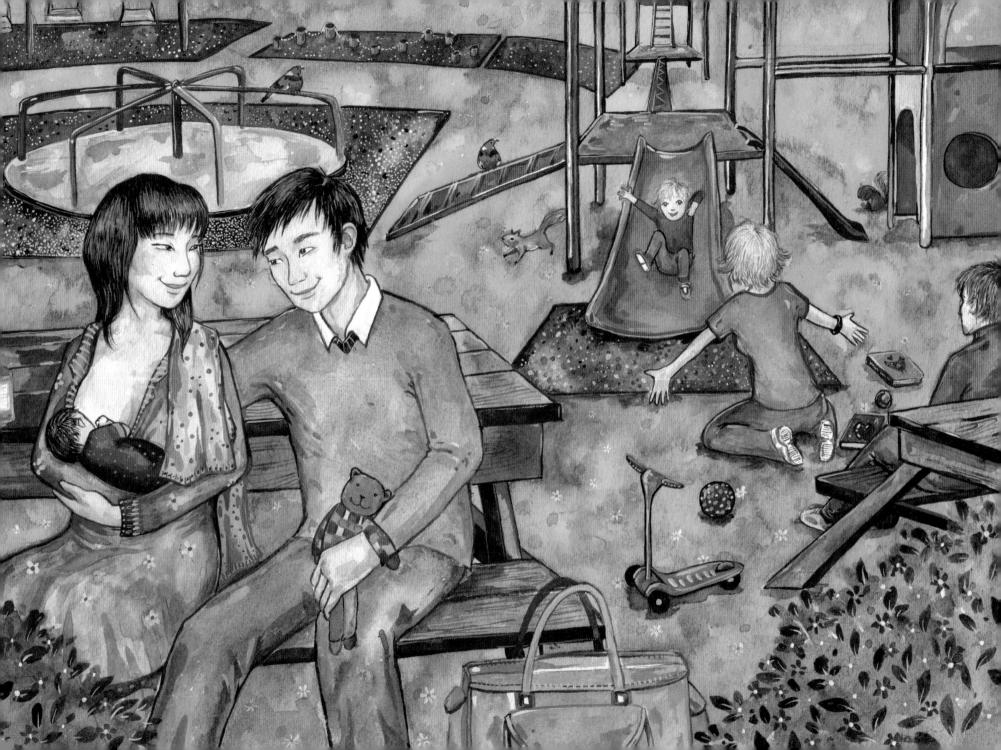

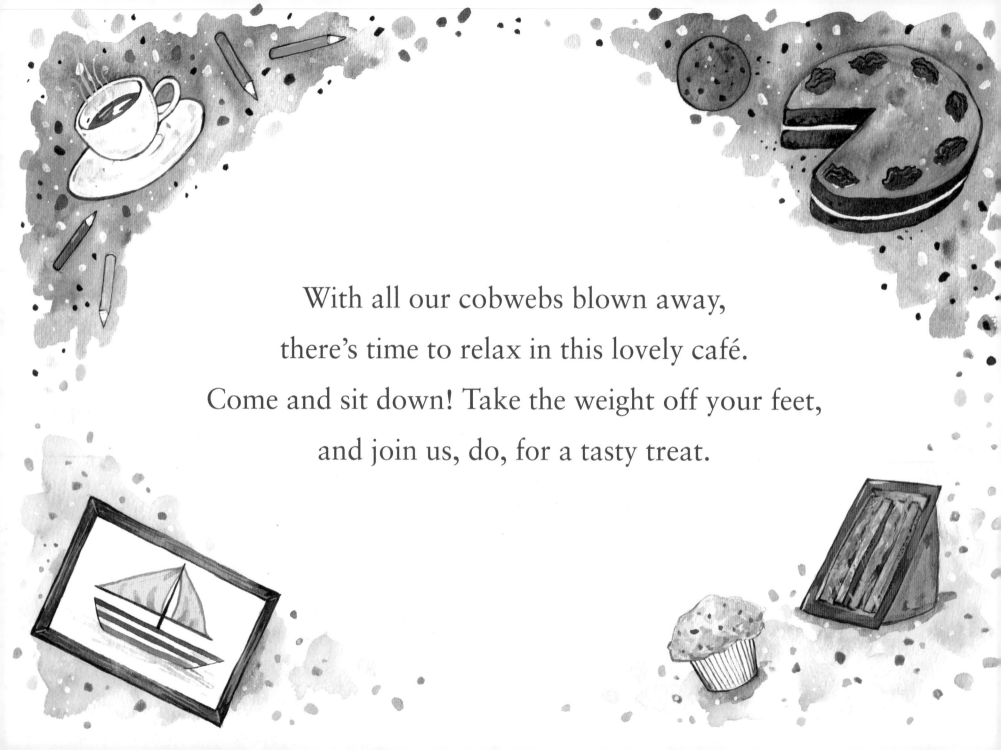

With all our cobwebs blown away,

there's time to relax in this lovely café.

Come and sit down! Take the weight off your feet,

and join us, do, for a tasty treat.

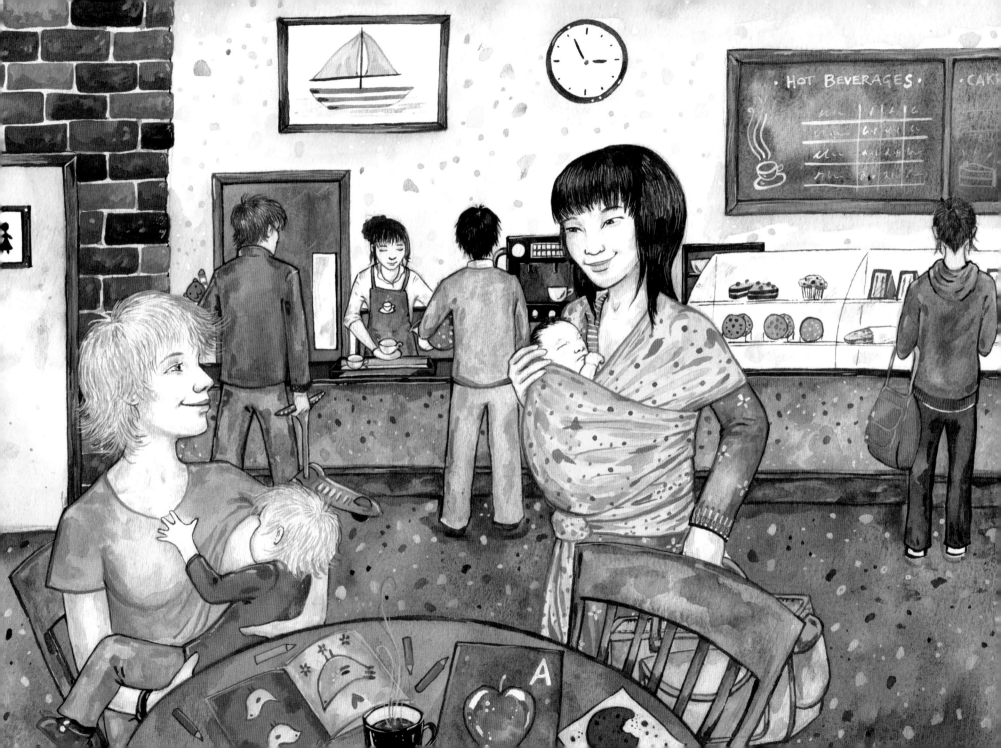

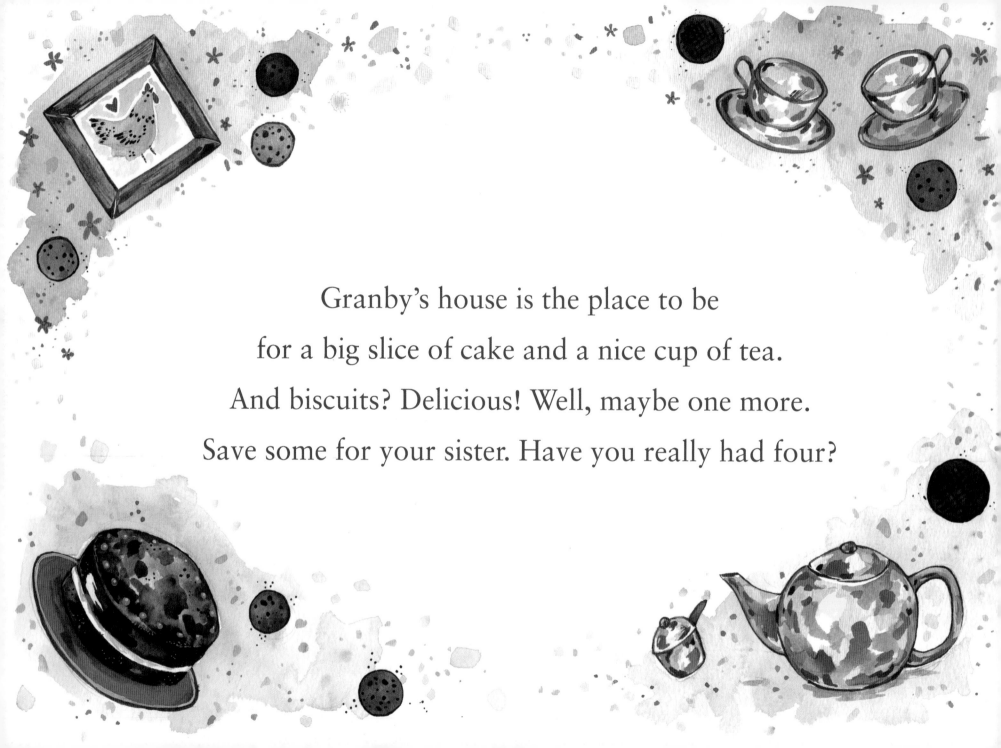

Granby's house is the place to be

for a big slice of cake and a nice cup of tea.

And biscuits? Delicious! Well, maybe one more.

Save some for your sister. Have you really had four?

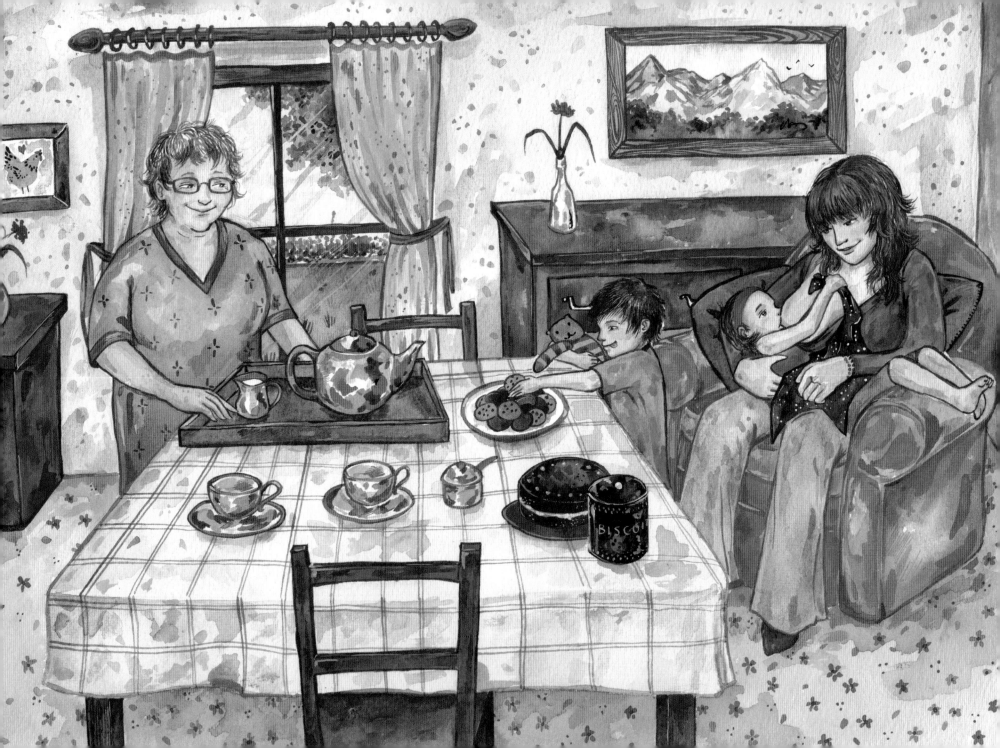

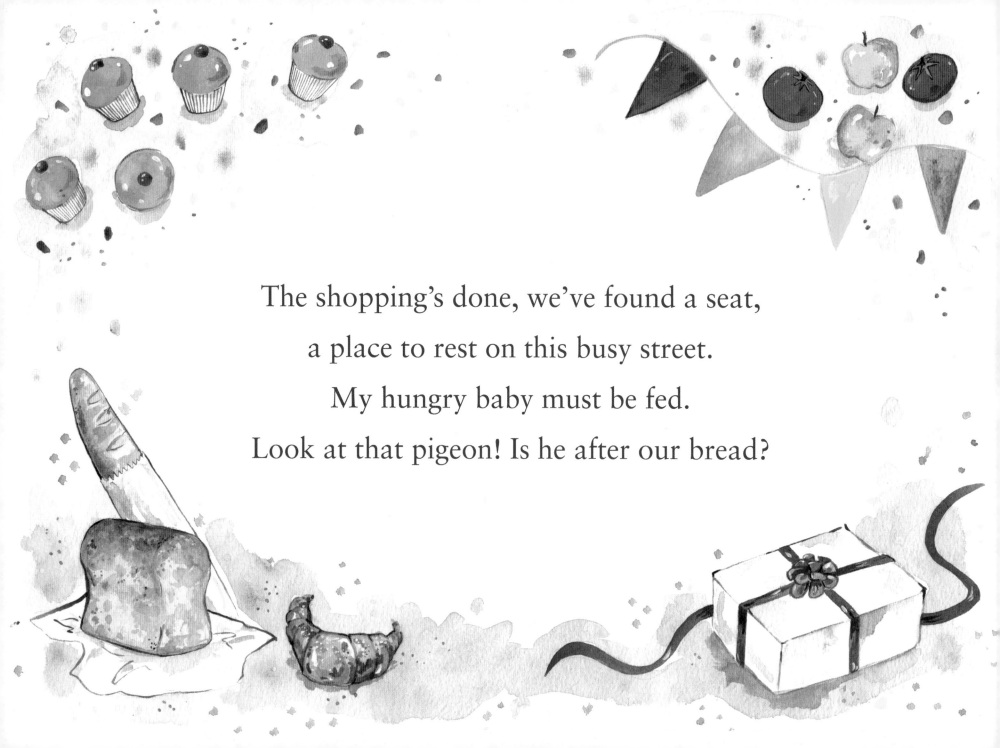

The shopping's done, we've found a seat,

a place to rest on this busy street.

My hungry baby must be fed.

Look at that pigeon! Is he after our bread?

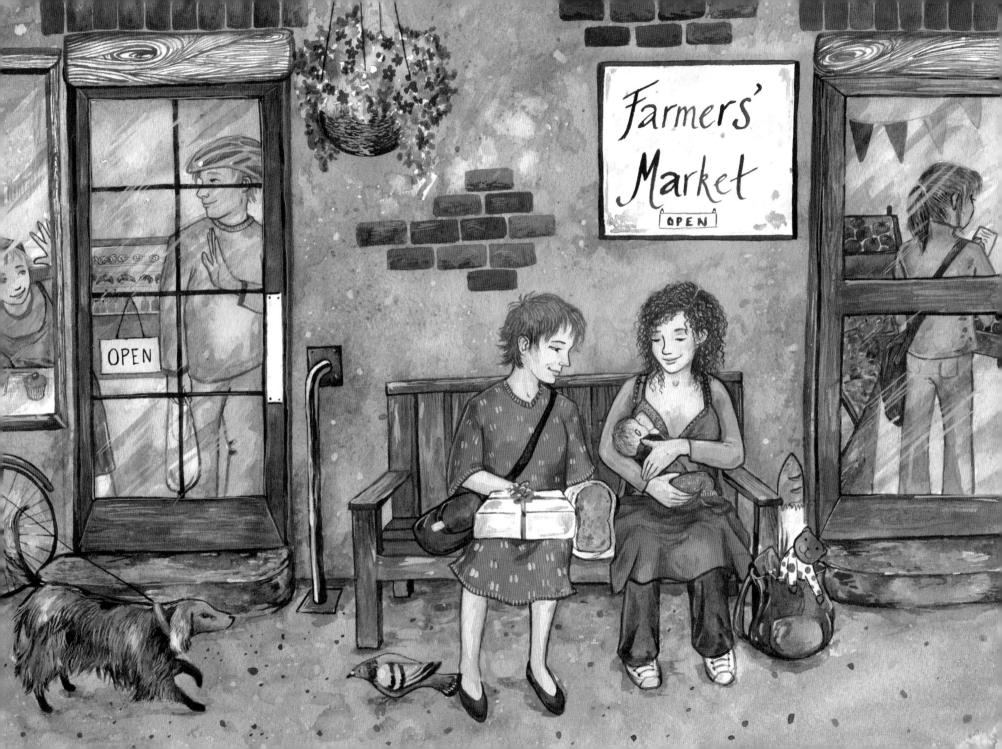

Farmers' Market

OPEN

OPEN

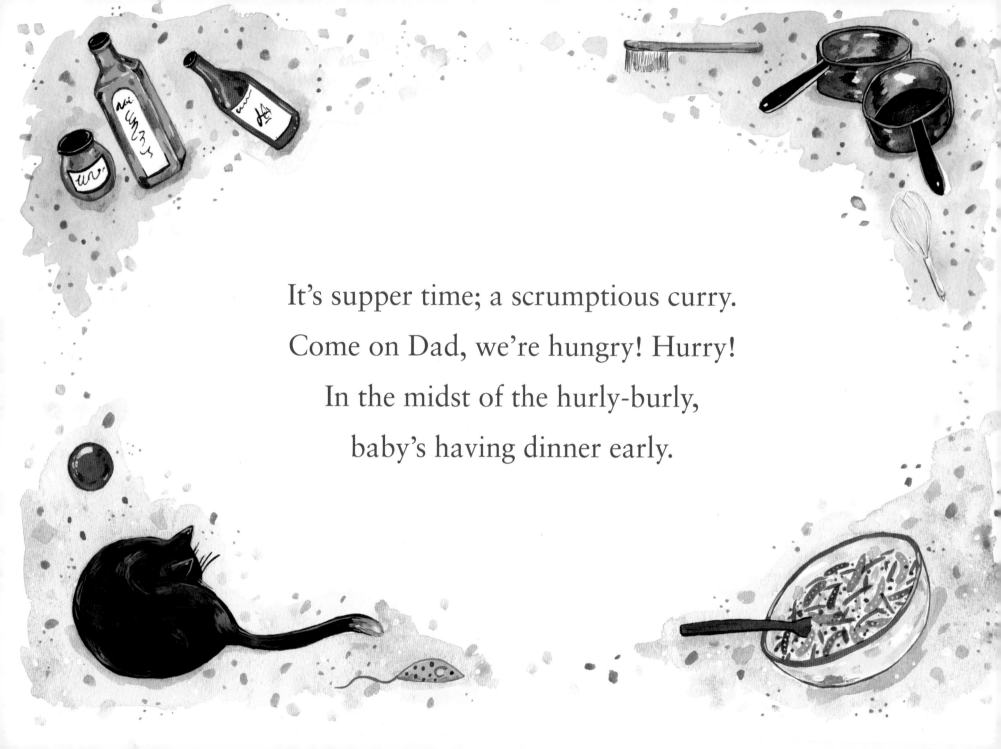

It's supper time; a scrumptious curry.

Come on Dad, we're hungry! Hurry!

In the midst of the hurly-burly,

baby's having dinner early.

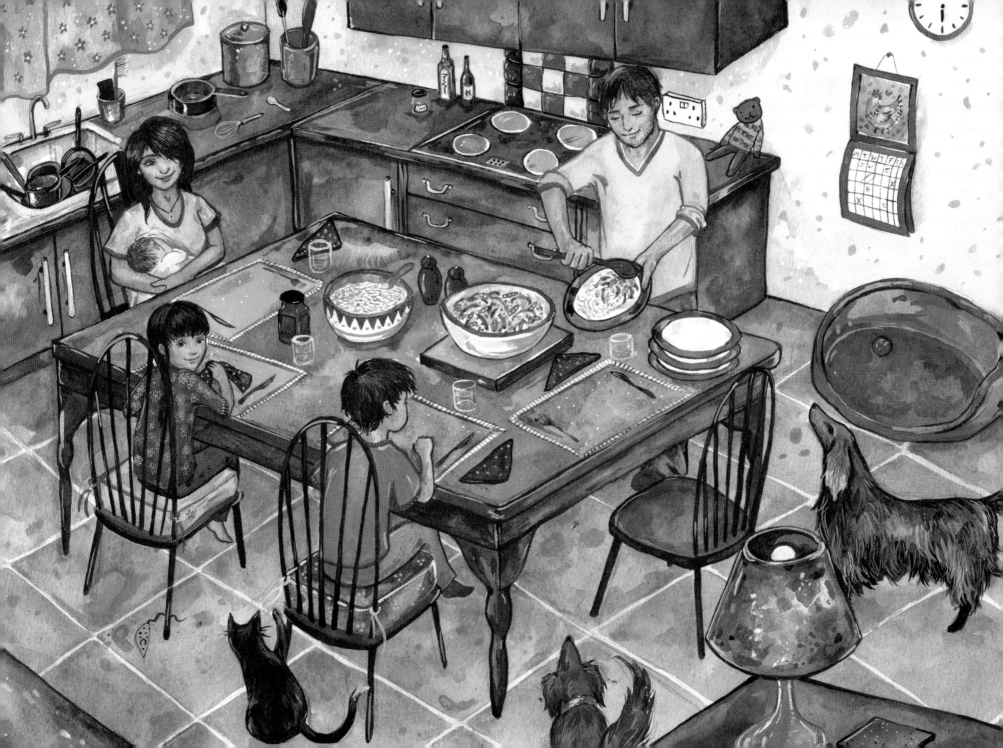

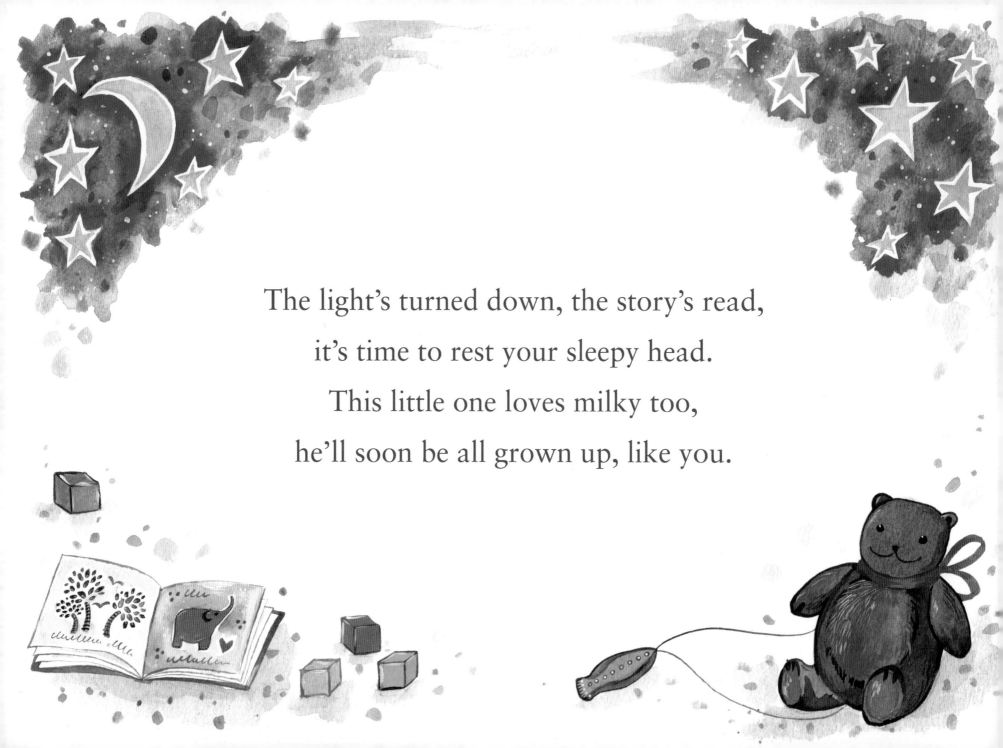

The light's turned down, the story's read,

it's time to rest your sleepy head.

This little one loves milky too,

he'll soon be all grown up, like you.

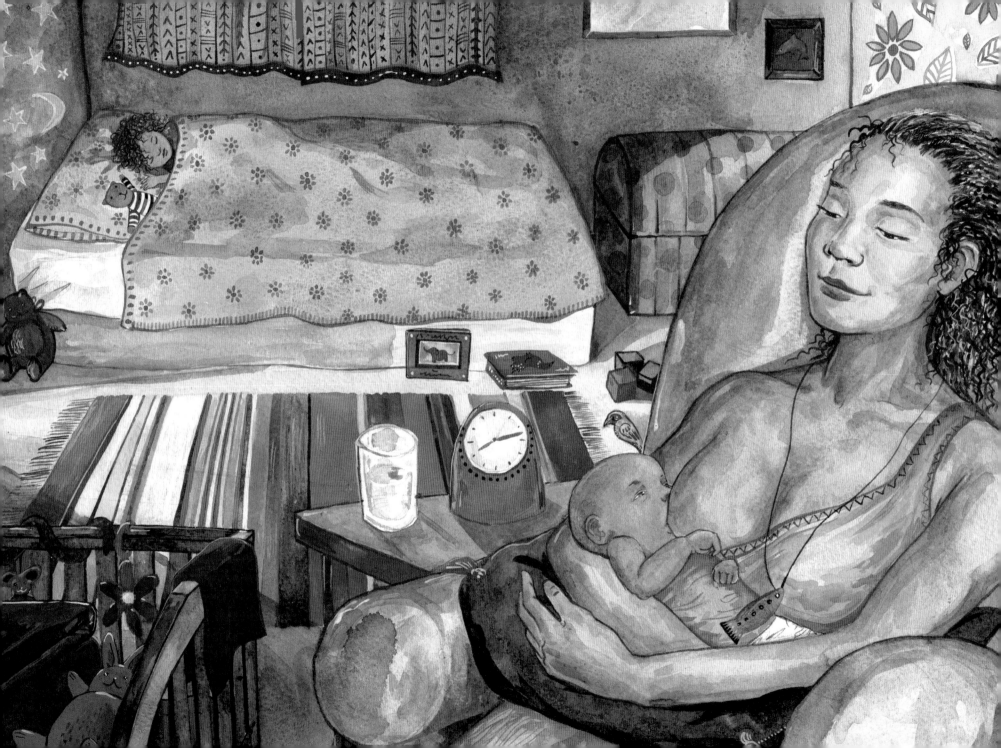

Here are the families! Now take a look:
see if you can find where they are in the book!

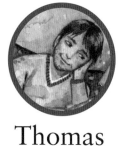 Maya

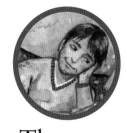 Thomas

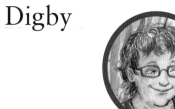 Ruth

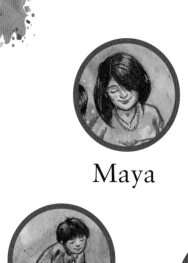 Alexander

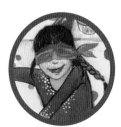 Lorenzo

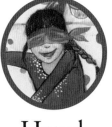 Hazel

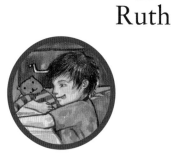 Digby

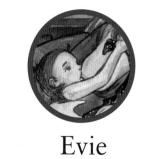 Evie

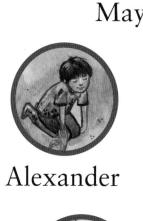 Holly

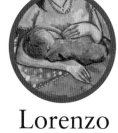 Maizie

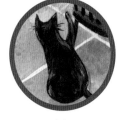 Wilbur

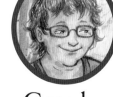 Granby

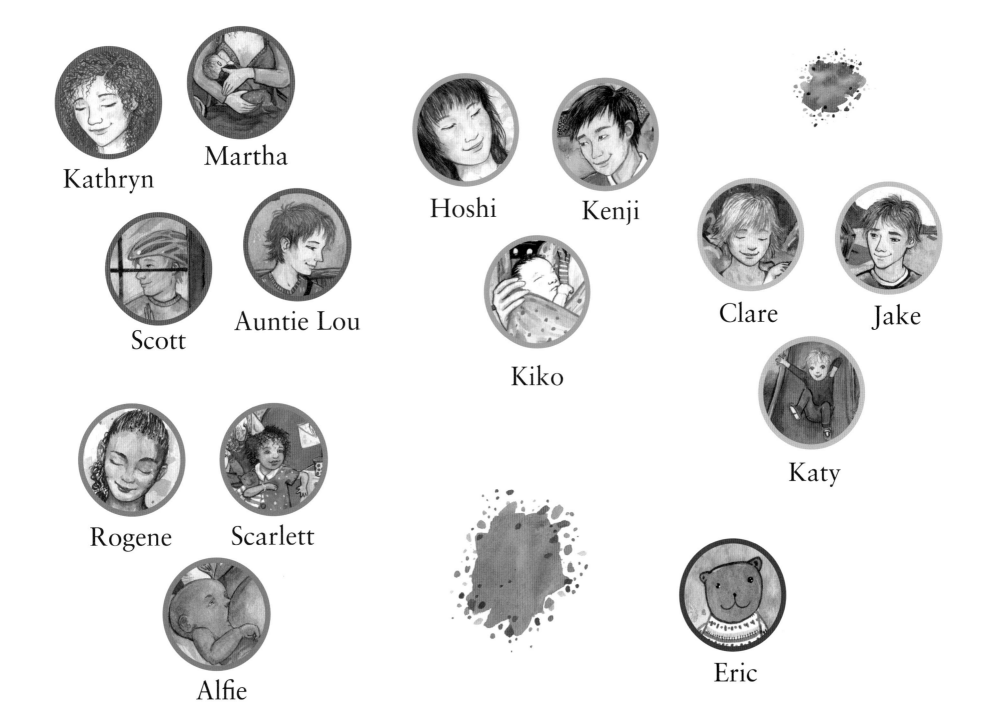

Kathryn

Martha

Scott

Auntie Lou

Hoshi

Kenji

Kiko

Clare

Jake

Katy

Rogene

Scarlett

Alfie

Eric

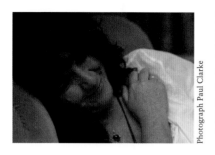

Photograph Paul Clarke

Ellie Stoneley gave birth to her daughter at the age of 47 and three years later they are still enjoying breastfeeding. When she's not writing or singing songs about scarecrows and black sheep with toddlers, Ellie works freelance helping small charities and businesses. She studied Psychology and English Literature, and has worked all over the world, most notably mining opals in the Australian outback and reporting, as a volunteer, on the work of the Kitchen Table Charities Trust in Madagascar. Ellie writes regularly about mothering and being an older first-time mother on her blog Mush Brained Ramblings, and at Huffington Post, MumsNet, Mothering in the Middle, What to Expect and Breastfeeding Matters. She has appeared on TV and radio to discuss a variety of parenting issues.

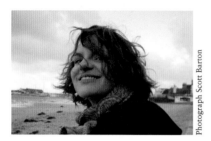

Photograph Scott Barton

Jessica began illustrating children's books in 2011 after having a go at studying everything from film production to veterinary medicine. After a few years of travelling and working, she sat down and started drawing chickens, which made her smile and, apparently, a lot of other people too. She has worked on several children's book covers as well as on various projects of her own, painting and creating stories alongside her fine art exhibitions. She is currently based, along with six chickens and a particularly friendly bonsai tree, in Cambridge, UK.

Share your milky moments at facebook.com/MilkyMomentsBook

For breastfeeding support contact La Leche League in the UK, the US and around the world.
laleche.org.uk | llli.org

also from Pinter & Martin

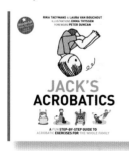
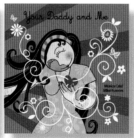
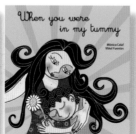
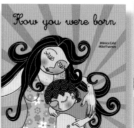
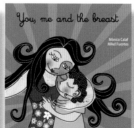
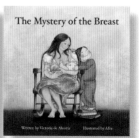

pinterandmartin.com